DAUGHTERS *Of* DEMENTIA

DAUGHTERS *Of* DEMENTIA

LESLIE BIRKLAND
LINDSEY DENHOF

Copyright © 2018 by Leslie Birkland

All rights reserved. No part of this book may be reproduced or transmitted in any form or by any means, electronic or mechanical, including photocopying, recording, or by any information storage and retrieval system, except in the case of brief quotations embodied in critical articles and reviews, without prior written permission of the publisher.

ISBN Paperbacl: 978-1717539397

Printed in the United States of America

Interior design: Ghislain Viau

*To our dear mother, Judith Denhof.
We witnessed the sadness of her heartache and the
strength of her perseverance, and have learned so
much from her. Her unwavering faith in the Lord
kept us all together throughout this journey.*

CONTENTS

Introduction		...1
CHAPTER 1	Mom Gets Married – Leslie	3
CHAPTER 2	Dad In a Nutshell – Lindsey	9
CHAPTER 3	Life With Dad – Lindsey	13
CHAPTER 4	Gone Goofy – Lindsey	19
CHAPTER 5	Men And Their Cars – Leslie	25
CHAPTER 6	The Reunion – Leslie	29
CHAPTER 7	Snow Day – Lindsey	35
CHAPTER 8	Showdown at the Bella Villa – Leslie	43
CHAPTER 9	Cheater – Leslie	51
CHAPTER 10	The Day My Dad Forgot Me – Lindsey	55
CHAPTER 11	Breaking News – Leslie	61
CHAPTER 12	Diaper Duty – Leslie	67
CHAPTER 13	Support Groups – Leslie	73

CHAPTER 14 | Hospice – Leslie 77
CHAPTER 15 | The Day My Dad Died
– Lindsey. 83
CHAPTER 16 | Friends of Dementia – Leslie. . . . 85
CHAPTER 17 | Imagine – Leslie. 89
CHAPTER 18 | Dementia or Just
Getting Old – Leslie 93
About the Authors. 99

INTRODUCTION

Leslie and Lindsey are sisters who felt compelled to share personal and revealing stories about their father, Duane, as he fell deeper and deeper into the tragic, memory-robbing abyss called dementia. Lindsey remembers the day her father forgot who she was and the heartbreaking impact her father's dementia had on her. Leslie shares a significant number of similar heartbreaking moments. Dementia is not for the faint of heart.

The two sisters narrate their experiences born from different perspectives, but very much driven from the same heart—the heart of a daughter; Lindsey is Duane's biological daughter, and Leslie is his stepdaughter. They both share a great love for their father, and a similar grief for the loss they all experienced long before their father died. The sisters harbor hopes that, through sharing their stories about caring for a loved one battling dementia, their experience will resonate with others in a similar situation.

Their message is simple: "You are not alone in this journey. It is not your fault. Dementia does not discriminate, and it is NOT personal."

CHAPTER ONE

MOM GETS MARRIED – LESLIE

When my parents divorced, our mom pulled up her bootstraps and headed back to college. It was apparent to her that she needed a degree to support my big brother, Chris, and myself.

Going to college became the next step in a new phase of life if there was to be any sort of moving on. And, Mom was never the kind of woman to allow stagnation, even following a divorce. As painful as the ordeal was, it just couldn't end there, and our mom knew that well enough. Getting a good job and

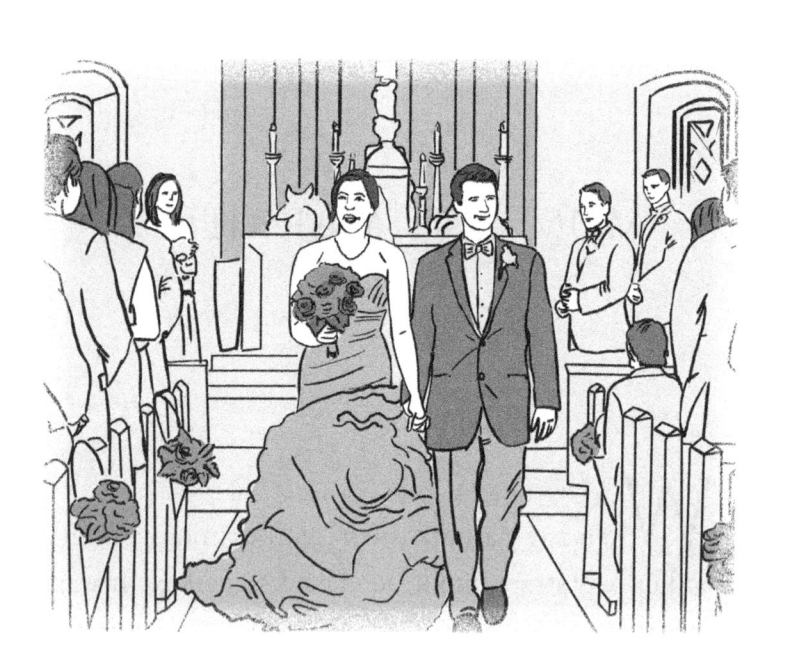

Mom Gets Married

getting us off welfare was a priority, while marrying again was the furthest thought from her mind.

Well, so she believed and repeated constantly, until she unexpectedly met Duane.

Duane was an old-school advertising executive. He was the Darrin Stephens (from the classic TV show *Bewitched*) of advertising. He also brought with him unique musical skills. He could play any tune on the piano *by ear*. He could write jingles in seconds, and his improvisations were hilarious. Duane, we all agreed, was the kind of man any woman would consider to be a perfect ten.

Duane was also quite dapper and drove a Mercedes. I had never been in a Mercedes before. Mom dearly loved to laugh, and Duane was a funny man. He brought out her laughter in full measure. This Mercedes-driving fox stole her heart through humor and just being an all-around great guy.

He was perfect, and they were perfect for each other. Their relationship seemed completely right. But nothing in life is entirely perfect. Duane had one little teeny flaw. He was not a Christian. He was not a member of any conflicting religion; he was simply not a Christian. For some women, that wouldn't have been a problem, but for Mom—a woman of deep faith—it was a massive issue.

"He is not a Christian," I can recall her saying with a tone of disbelief and slight hurt. Mom shared her faith with Duane, and it wasn't long before he accepted Jesus Christ as his Lord and Savior. A year later, they married at my family's church, where my uncle was the pastor.

In an exciting tone that still rings in my head, she had asked me, "Will you be my maid of honor?"

I remember how nervous and shy I was, but I wanted to make Mom happy and agreed to be part of the wedding. I made my own dress for the ceremony. It was a turquoise-blue halter gown with boa trim. Perhaps not entirely appropriate for a wedding, but I loved it, Mom approved of it, and that's all that mattered.

I made most of my clothes back in those days. We didn't have enough money to throw around like the wealthy kids would, so if I wanted to stay in fashion—and I did—I had no other choice but to learn how to sew. Fortunately, I loved sewing and was good at it, too.

I remember window shopping at Nordstrom, thinking, *One day I will be able to shop here.*

I also had dreams of becoming a model. At age sixteen, Duane recommended me to a client for my first modeling job. I must have done a pretty good job for this client because he hired me a few more times. Duane was always positive and encouraged me to pursue my modeling dreams. Who knew then, that I would ultimately become a model for Nordstrom?

CHAPTER TWO

DAD IN A NUTSHELL – LINDSEY

With his affable personality and ready smile, I doubt there was the slightest possibility that Dad was disliked by anyone. In truth, I know of no one who disliked him, and I can't imagine that anyone would speak badly about the man.

Duane Denhof, the provider of jests and jokes, always filled a room with smiles and laughter. My memory contains nothing but recollections of a kind, gentle man. Never once do I recall hurtful criticism or harmful belittling. Dad was a genuinely nice and supportive person.

He was also incredibly funny with an original sense of humor. One day he discovered my mother holding a statue of a small frog. My mother and I had come across the statue while wandering the aisles of Uwajimaya, a popular Asian market in downtown Seattle. To our delight, the amphibious merchandise elicited one of his witticisms. "What we have here is a Ribbit Exhibit," he said, offering up for posterity one of our favorite Duane-isms—clever, eye-rolling jokes that Mom and I would repeat over and over.

Looking back now, I realize I often find myself saying things exactly the way Dad did. Recently, a nun visited my workplace. Making a small misstep, she nearly knocked over one of my supervisors, and a perfect example of how I mimic my dad just popped out of my mouth:

"Better tell her not to make it a habit!" I said, before gasping in shock and realization, while my hands clamped against my mouth. *God! That was so Dad!*

My hesitation and fervent desire not to emulate him stemmed from the fact that I had often viewed his humor as cheesy. I was slightly hesitant to admit that I had inherited that trait! I appreciate that this form of comedy is a display of the creative process, though, and I have come to value and miss it now that he is gone.

I sit here, studying an old picture of my family. I look to be a toddler; mom and dad sitting in front, while my brother and sister stand directly behind them. My brother, with a happy smile across his face, is holding me. Mom's gaze is fixed on the person behind the camera, while Dad has a different kind of look across his face—neither a smile, nor a frown.

In the picture, he looks vague and dream-like, and his expression is hard to discern. It makes me wonder if he was experiencing the moment as the rest of us were. Mom believes that Dad was showing signs of his dementia many years prior to being diagnosed.

Studying the photograph today, I cannot help but wonder if he was experiencing just a hint of what was to come while none of us knew anything about it, blissfully unaware of what was to be.

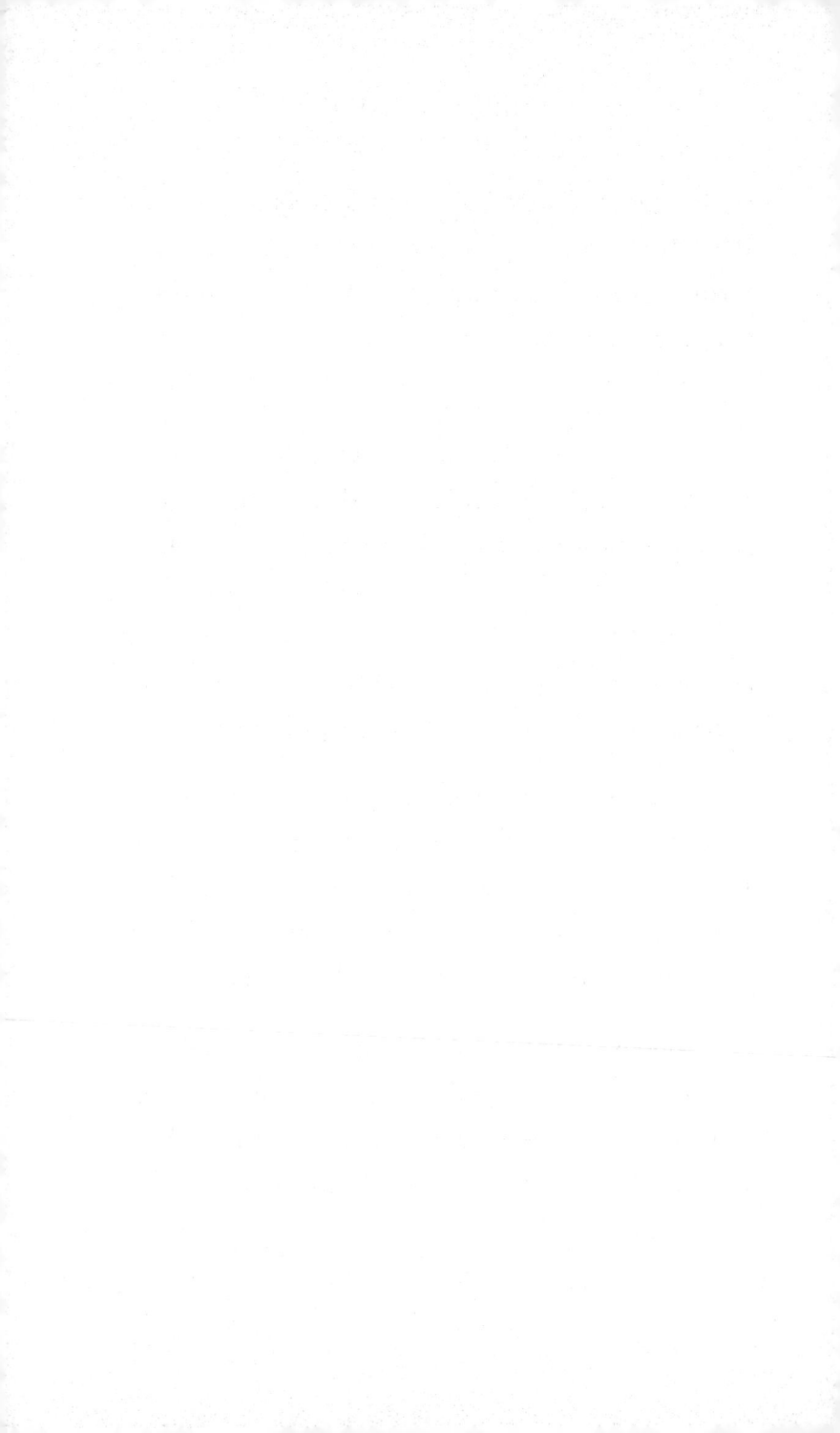

CHAPTER THREE

LIFE WITH DAD – LINDSEY

I counted myself rather fortunate because I had my parents all to myself; my older brother and sister were out of the house enjoying their own families and careers, while I settled in as the sole child they were responsible for day-in-day-out in close proximity. It was an experience I cherished and often still find myself thinking about how lucky I had been.

A few years after I was born, Mom quit her job to become a stay-at-home parent. At the same time, Dad created an office in the house. That meant he was home most of the time and was willing and

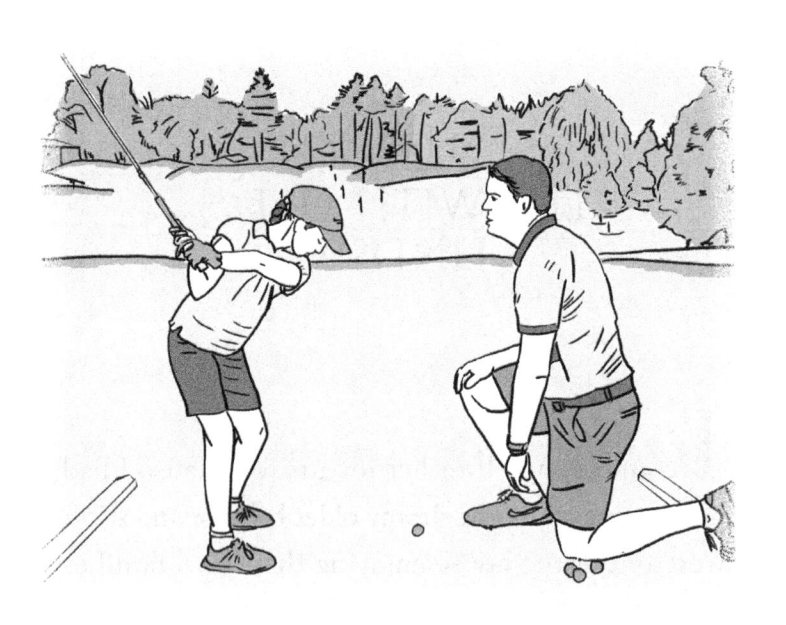

Life With Dad

able to lend a supporting hand to things around the house. I attended a private Christian school, and for all intents and purposes, I can proudly say I had the perfect upbringing.

Dad and I shared an interest in sports. Although I was little, I excelled at baseball and golf. Dad was my biggest fan and my first golf coach. I got so good at the sport that Mom and Dad decided to hire a pro to take over my coaching. I competed in golf tournaments throughout Washington State. By the time I was twelve, I ranked second in the state, which at the time wasn't that big of a deal to me. It was simply something I enjoyed doing with my dad.

Dad had graduated from the University of Washington, so it was no surprise that he took me to every type of Husky sporting event. Our shared love of sports wasn't the only thing we had going on, because we also shared a love for music. The love for music is something I inherited from Dad. Even though Dad was completely deaf in one ear, he could play on the piano any song after hearing it only once. He was truly gifted with a special musical ability.

He shared that gift with me, for which I am so grateful. My love for music helped in developing my ability to compose music and play the guitar. I now mostly play at church or small venues and local coffee shops.

Where Dad really excelled was in his amazing sense of humor. Dad really was a funny fellow who always sought what was comical in any situation he found himself or others around him in.

There is a saying that "Super funny people aren't entirely funny at home."

Dad was an exception, because he was able to entertain me all the time.

Dad and I would have long talks about life and the future. I was close enough to him to share almost anything. It way evident that mom was extremely joyous and had a sense of satisfaction when she recognized the bond and closeness dad and I shared.

He was not just my father, but my hero.

"I PLACED MY FATHER'S HANDS ON THE IVORY KEYS AND HE PROCEEDED TO PLAY LOUIE LOUIE WITH GUSTO."

—LINDSEY DENHOF

CHAPTER FOUR
GONE GOOFY – LINDSEY

Dementia didn't come quickly or with a loud bang and trumpet announcing its arrival. Instead, the signs of its entrance into our lives hung quietly over and around us, slowly trying to make its presence known for years. The first signs tricked themselves into our consciousness stealthily at first. There was no great line of demarcation. Certain things just didn't make sense. I mean, how was I or anyone meant to know those strange little quirks he was exhibiting had something to do with dementia?

"Let's go to the zoo!" he would say.

We did at one time live a few blocks from Woodland Park Zoo, but had moved years prior. That fact aside, he would announce the excited proposal to go to the zoo when I was no longer a kid. I was in college, and going to the zoo was nowhere near the list of thrilling things someone at my age wanted to spend hours of personal time doing. It didn't just end at asking us to go to the zoo, either, but his request also extended toward random strangers.

He would ask teenagers he met on the street if they were in one of his classes at the University of Washington. Other symptoms eased in slowly, indicating that Dad was finding it hard to learn new things or even keep a grasp on things he already knew very well. The ability to retain new information he had recently learned was slowly drifting away, and it seemed like he was living in the past, especially his college days.

For someone whose job demanded and required that he keep himself abreast of the newest things and remain cutting-edge current on trends for the world of advertising, it became a big stumbling block, which we were yet to fully understand as the signs remained low key and under the surface.

Gone Goofy

He could clearly remember how to put a brochure together using out-of-date techniques, but he struggled to use the new ones being implemented by his peers. He would cut and paste photostats and text with an Exacto blade. Computers had been out for years, but he preferred the old layout style and stuck with it as technology passed him by. His inability to master technology affected his life in every possible way. It became a major threat when it began messing with his job.

One at a time, clients stopped calling for jobs to be done, and gradually, over time, there were none.

Sometimes, Dad would wander around the house wearing a mask of loss across his face, prompting questions from me in the process.

"Are you looking for something, Dad? Is there anything specific you are searching for?" I remember asking more than once.

I got the same answer every time. "I am looking for clues."

I often wondered whether he was joking or really looking for clues. I found the answer disturbing. I realize that he was indeed looking for clues; clues around the house that might give him an indication about what he was supposed to do.

Finally, Mom took him to a neurologist. I recall vividly the day Mom sat me down to share the diagnosis. "Your father has dementia. He has probably had it for some time."

I broke out in tears. My dad was drifting away, and it broke my heart to pieces.

> "IF YOU LEARN TO LISTEN FOR CLUES AS TO HOW I FEEL INSTEAD OF WHAT I SAY, YOU WILL BE ABLE TO UNDERSTAND ME BETTER."
>
> —MARA BOTONIS

CHAPTER FIVE

MEN AND THEIR CARS – LESLIE

Duane's diagnosis meant one thing: Mom had no choice but to go back to work. The first few months when Duane had to be at home by himself wasn't as bad as we'd thought it would be. In fact, he did considerably well, and it wasn't entirely worrisome. He could remember things like his name, where he lived, how to microwave a meal, and how to answer the phone. Provided it was something he had learned in the past, he could do it. In fact, he excelled in things he had known from his past and had no issues carrying them out routinely. He would spend hours upon hours walking to the Goodwill and buying old cassette tapes for 25 cents each. Then, he would spend days categorizing the cassette tapes as though he hoped to achieve something important from performing the task in the most careful way.

Once a week Mom would return the cassettes tapes back to the Goodwill, so Duane could repurchase them the following week. It was a cycle Mom indulged him in, and all I could do was watch in dismay.

He was still driving the car. "Why would you let him drive a car in his current state?" I asked once. One of the few times in my life I raised my voice to my mother.

Mom sighed and replied, "It is one of the few things he has left, and I cannot take it away from him."

I could understand what she was saying, but it still baffled me and I was forced to speak on.

"Yes, but what if he forgets how to drive? What if he forgets it while driving, or worse, he runs over a child?" There is a fine line between safety and maintaining the dignity of those we love, and we were right up against that line.

Mom held her ground. She knew that it was the last bit of his independence, and she couldn't bear to take that away from the man she loved.

I thought about it for a while and finally said, "Okay, if that's the case, I want you to promise me one thing, that at the funeral of the child he runs over, you will tell those parents that you couldn't bear to take the car keys away because it was the last bit of your husband's independence."

Mom took the car keys away that day and gave the car to one of her grandchildren. Fortunately, Duane was not the kind of guy who was attached to or identified his manliness with a car. He adjusted to his new situation with the calm humor he brought to the rest of his life.

CHAPTER SIX

THE REUNION – LESLIE

One of the most disturbing things about dementia is the fact that quite often the person inflicted with the disease finds himself appearing normal and sounding exactly the way every normal person would with no indication from his tone of voice or his actions that something unusual is happening.

The problem remains shielded as if in a mirage. For a long time, those close to people afflicted with dementia can easily deny or dismiss the condition, because it appears that nothing is really wrong. Their speech patterns remain very much the same, their actions seem no different, and they relate with those around them in a very natural, typical way. They can engage in lengthy, sensible, and intellectual conversations, although there are certain aspects that may be lacking, but they're subtle and might not be seen even by those with an observant eye. These small changes may include the inability to know what year or day it is, but they can maintain the semblance of normalcy. It simply means many people who are unaware of the diagnosis might not know the person has dementia if the sufferer's symptoms are not yet profound.

Mom, for whatever reason, did not tell many people about Duane's dementia. He looked great and talked a good talk, so why share her burden or embarrassment? I tried times without count to convince Mom to share the situation of his diagnosis with people so they could know, especially the neighbors, but she declined on every turn, and I slowly began to forbid myself from asking.

If he had cancer, would that embarrass her too? I had thought at times, and tried hard not to ask Mom so I wouldn't come across as rude. It wasn't his fault, or anybody's fault, that he had a disease, and he needed

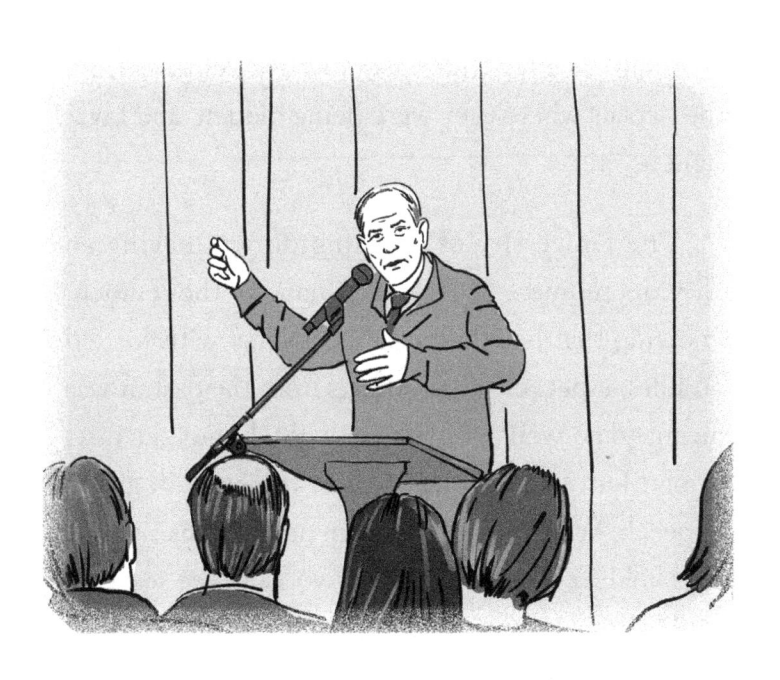

understanding from the people around him. Who knows what crazy, convincing tales he could tell the neighborhood?

I had a feeling things would slowly emerge from the depths where they were being hidden, and I was right as rain.

The University of Washington was having an all-years reunion. Mom took Duane to the reunion, knowing that he could easily converse with his old buddies, especially about things from the past. It was meant to go well and without a glitch, but the next thing Mom knew, Duane was at the podium giving a speech. With hearts beating in our mouths and our eyes holding so much fear and worry in the seats we could barely contain ourselves in, Mom and I prayed fervently for him not to make a mess of things.

Surprisingly, it turned out to be a wonderful, thought provoking, and inspirational speech about what he had accomplished since his college days. He spoke of his involvement in philanthropy, his church, and his travels all over the world. It was a beautiful, award-winning speech. Mom sat there in utter amazement as his friends and former colleagues applauded. The only problem was, *not one word was true.* Mom knew that this altered state of reality was part of the illness, but goodness, this sure was a doozy.

CHAPTER SEVEN

SNOW DAY – LINDSEY

It wasn't as if we didn't predict it or as though it wasn't a worry of mine that I held close to my heart and constantly prayed and feared it might come to be when we weren't expecting it. It haunted me. In all honesty, being introduced to the world of dementia because someone close to me was going through it brought a degree of enlightenment I never could have expected.

It also brought the feeling that the shoe was waiting to drop.

The day finally came when Dad was unable to make it home without help.

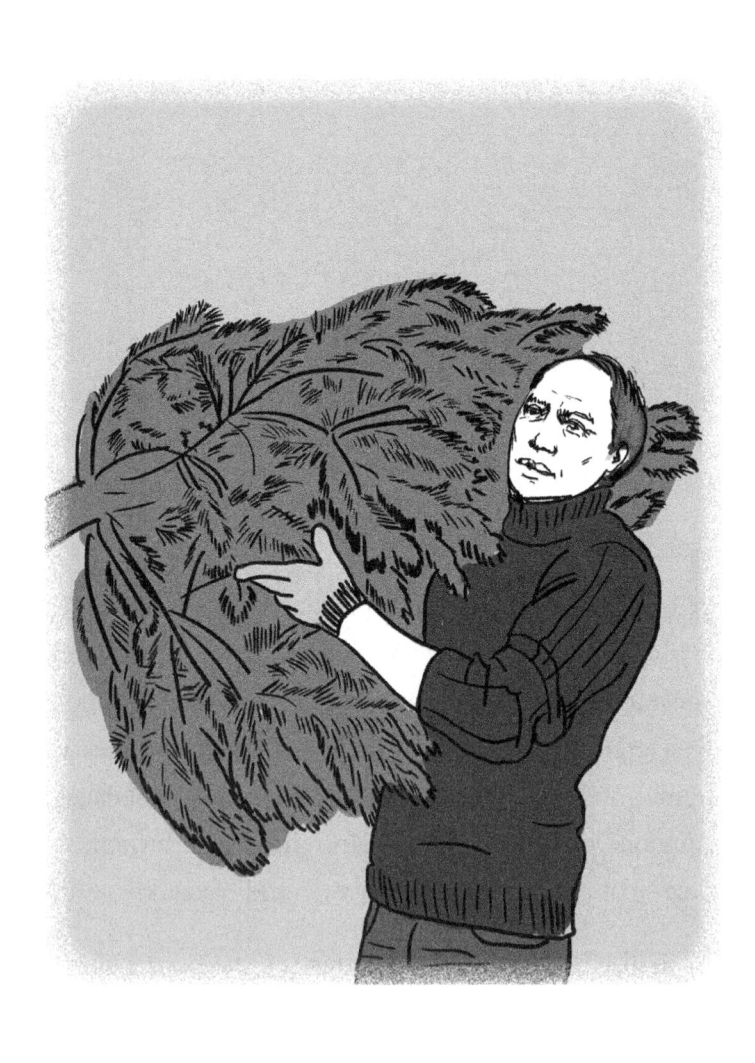

Snow Day

Mom arrived home from work one day, and did not recognize her house. *Oh, it looks nice*, she must have thought, with just one major problem accompanying the new look.

It just so disturbingly happened that everything in the house had been reorganized to new and sometimes unusual locations. Two weeks before Christmas, Duane had taken down the Christmas tree and carefully put all the ornaments away. He didn't stop there. He went ahead and opened all the presents and put them away too, with the exception of a nice pair of Gloria Vanderbilt jeans, which fit him nicely, by the way, if I may say so.

So much for surprising Mom with what I got her this year, I thought and sighed with exhaustion.

Mom was visibly displeased. She was displeased for a host of reasons, and not only because of what he had done, but I think also because Dad was able to fit into her jeans. Between my sister Leslie and I, we came up with a somewhat workable schedule to insure he couldn't get into too much trouble while Mom was at work. It was the best we could do considering the circumstances.

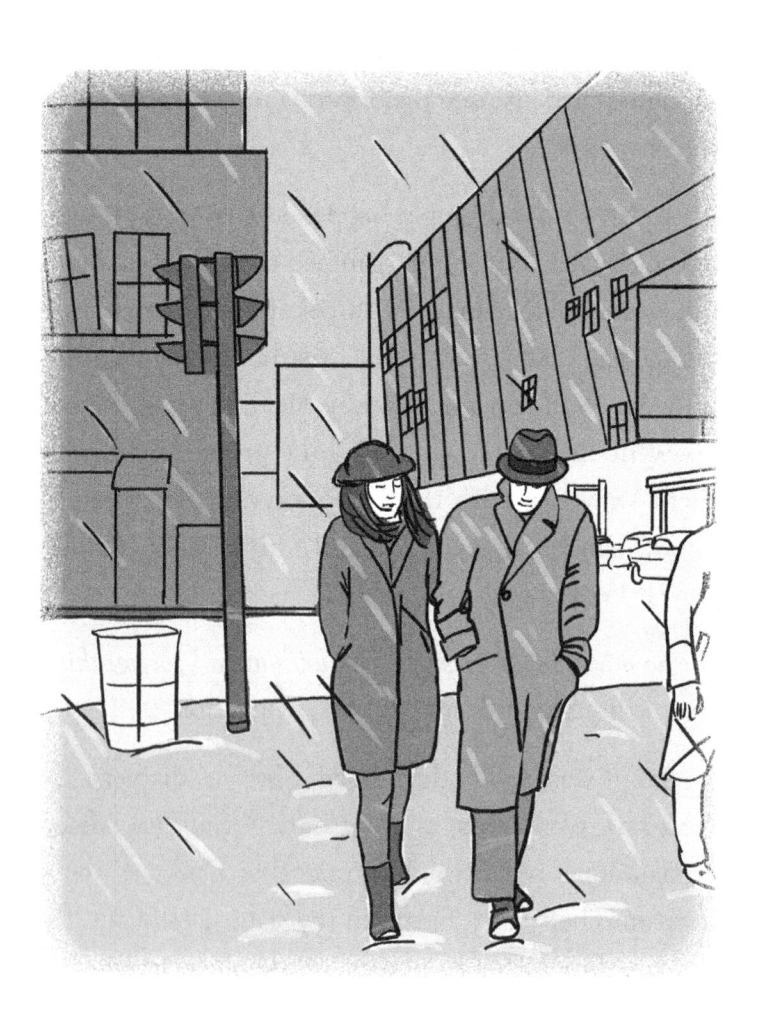

Snow Day

One snowy afternoon, I decided to take Dad for a stroll. He needed to get out of the house, and so did I. Soon, the light snow became a snowstorm, and cars were beginning to slide around. It was time to take Dad back home.

Dad was walking one pace behind me. I looked back, and he was gone. "Where is he?" I asked myself and panicked.

It was baffling and disturbing. My heart began to thud endlessly against my rib cage in hurt and worry as I searched around for the man to no avail.

I soon admitted to myself that I had lost my dad. I yelled for him, but he did not answer. I retraced our steps about thirty yards before I saw him. And there he was in the middle of the street, directing traffic. Oddly enough he was doing a pretty good job and drivers were following his directions, but that did nothing to relieve my anxiety.

"For the love of God, Dad, please get over here!" I yelled.

He looked at me without the slightest sign of recognition and said, "Can I help you, Sir?"

"I'm your daughter! And we are going home," I fumed.

"TO CARE FOR THOSE WHO CARED FOR US IS ONE OF THE HIGHEST HONORS."

—TIA WALKER

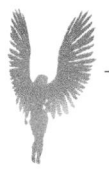

CHAPTER EIGHT

SHOWDOWN AT THE BELLA VILLA – LESLIE

Mom and Duane moved to a new place to be closer to me. Lindsey moved back in with Mom and Duane to better assist Mom. I helped Mom fill out the lease agreement. Her biggest fear was that the manager would find out that Duane had dementia and would not allow them to move in. It wasn't news to us that some people believed that those with dementia were dangerous or crazy and didn't exactly welcome them in their buildings. I suppose they thought patients with dementia were lunatics; obviously they had no experience with the disease or the people affected.

What I realized was that the stress of having to find a suitable place for my parents to stay wasn't one my Mom was willing to put herself through. I wasn't ready for it either.

"We'll keep him safe and away from prying eyes . . . whatever it takes," she said in confidence and with a hint of emotion in her voice.

The Bella Villa complex was large, and Mom thought no one would pay much attention to them in there, which made it even more perfect considering the circumstances surrounding their situation. We set the plan in place, and everything looked perfect until the day arrived for Mom, Lindsey, and Duane to officially move in. Things got a little hectic.

Without our being aware, Duane decided to take a shower.

As we were carrying boxes into the apartment, we all heard a disturbingly loud scream. Dropping everything, we raced toward the terrified sound of Duane's voice calling for help and discovered that Duane had forgotten how to take a shower. The temperature of the water was nearly scalding. He was half dressed, soaking wet, and had emptied an entire bottle of shampoo on his face, in his eyes and on the floor. The shampoo in his eyes obviously stung him, and his response was to scream and cry out loud like a child who wanted his mother to come to his aid.

She wept endlessly.

"Forgot how" is a common thing with dementia. One moment you can throw a ball, and the next moment you can't say ball, let alone remember what to do with it. Unlike the movie *The Notebook*, once something is forgotten, it's unlikely to return. Duane soon started a routine of walking in circles. He would do hours of circles in a baffling and disturbing manner from the kitchen to the hallway and back to the kitchen again.

One time, in a moment of frustration Mom yelled, "What are you doing?"

I understood better than she did at that point in time, and I explained to Mom.

"Each circle he makes around is the first circle for him," I said.

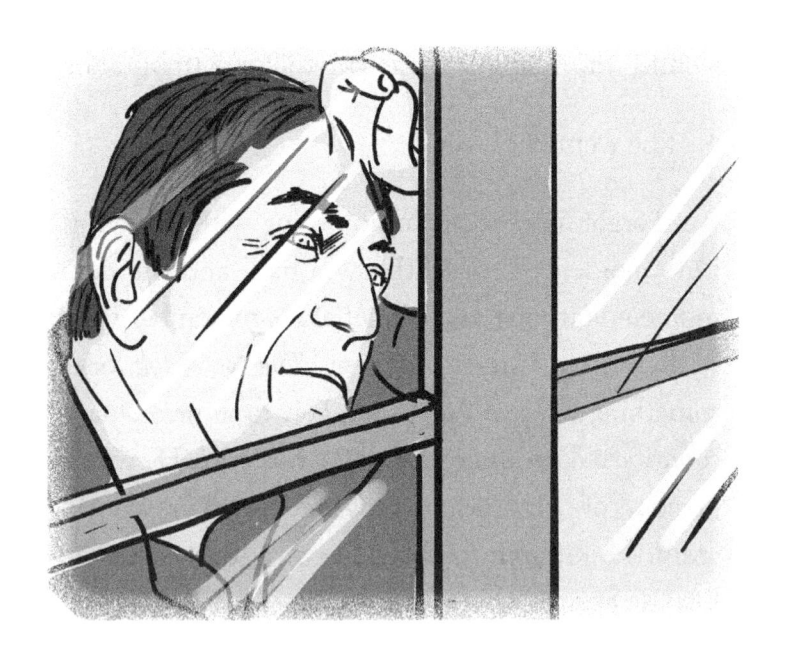

Showdown at the Bella Villa

About three months later, the apartment manager called me for an impromptu meeting. I had no understanding what it would be about, but I was curious to find out. She was a lovely young gal in her twenties. In the nicest possible way she told me that people were complaining about Duane. I felt I should have thought of it sooner, but we had managed to keep him in check, or at least I thought we had contained him. I did not realize Duane had somehow found a way to terrify people around the complex.

I found out from the manager we weren't doing the awesome job I thought we were doing.

"Kids are scared of him, and some of the residents have even threatened to move," she explained with a pained face.

Apparently, during the times Mom was at work or running an errand, Duane would open the window and close the window over and over and over in a repetitive and quite disturbing manner.

"He tells neighbors he has to get home to Canada and that he needs a ride, or he'll simply hop in their car." The apartment manager recounted my dad's actions further, and though they were abnormal for the Duane we used to know, they were sounding like something he definitely could do now.

I had no way of defending him or denying the offenses laid before me. All I could do was sit and listen with my hands between my thighs.

She continued, "He opened and shut the front door every 10 seconds, for hours."

I was stuck on what to do or say, and I finally decided to go against Mom's wishes and flat out said, "Duane has dementia."

I will never forget her response. She said, "Stop. Say no more. I get it."

The residents soon found a special place in their hearts for Duane and treated him with kindness and understanding from that point on. In fact they kind of looked after him once they became aware of his illness. It is critical that people around us are aware if someone has dementia. It can be dangerous for the person afflicted and also for the people unaware of the situation. For example, people with dementia may innocently walk into a stranger's home or hop into their cars. It is not normal behavior for people to do this, and it would be within someone's rights to defend himself or his family. In fact I believe there comes a time when it is negligent on the caregiver's part to not share this information with community members who live near, or are in contact with, the family.

Mom forgave me for spilling the beans with the apartment manager regarding Duane's condition. Mom soon came to the realization that people knowing about his illness is not a reflection of the man he once was or diminishes him in any fashion. In fact, Mom realized that most people are very compassionate once they have clarity.

CHAPTER NINE
CHEATER – LESLIE

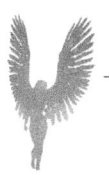

Sunday was my day for church, fellowship, and much-needed relaxation. On one particular Sunday, I remember hoping that this day would be just like any other Sunday before, but it was bound to be different. It was really early in the morning when I received a frantic call from Mom.

I recall watching the phone ring tirelessly and not picking it up immediately because I feared it was probably something about Duane. I was exhausted, and selfishly wanted one more hour of peace.

All I could think was, *Oh no, what now?*

Daughters of Dementia

With the last ounce of courage in me, knowing that the call had to do with Duane, I picked up the phone and slowly placed it against my ear with my lips refusing to speak immediately.

"Duane is cheating on me!!!!" Mom screamed.

Surely she must be joking, I thought immediately.

"Mom, I'm pretty sure Duane is NOT cheating on you," I replied as calmly as I could.

Mom insisted that it was true, and the tone of her voice was convincing me as well.

"Okay, Mom, so who is the other woman with whom he is cheating?" I had to ask.

"ME!" she said.

I was temporarily lost, pondering whether I had heard her correctly.

"Okay, so let me get this straight, Duane is cheating on you with you?" I asked.

"YES! I woke up this morning, and Duane told me I had to get out because his daughter was going to be home soon. I told him I was his wife, and he said,

Cheater

'Yeah, lady, try to pull that one over on me.' I left the room to gather my thoughts, and when I returned he saw me as Judi, his wife, and had a real guilty look on his face," she narrated perfectly.

Next came the question I knew I would regret, but I had to ask. I asked Mom if she and Duane were still romantic.

"Well, of course, dear. He is still a man." She ached the words into my ears.

I did some quick reasoning in my head and gave her a simple explanation as to what I thought had transpired. I told her that he went to bed with her, Judi, his wife, that night and woke to a woman he did not recognize. So essentially he did not cheat.

That scenario seemed to satisfy her, although I don't think she ever trusted his cheating ways again.

Dementia is horrible, horrible for everyone associated. But, I always said that there are times when one has to laugh, even a sad uncomfortable laugh, like in this case. Because if you don't laugh, you'd just be crying all day.

CHAPTER TEN

THE DAY MY DAD FORGOT ME – LINDSEY

This fateful day, Mom was at work and I had the day off. I had agreed to babysit Dad for the entire day. Before he woke up, I prepared our breakfast, and then we enjoyed a nice meal together.

For the umpteenth time, he was wearing Mom's Gloria Vanderbilt jeans again and a nice red turtleneck sweater, but what the heck, he looked nice. Then the unthinkable happened. Dad forgot me. It was not like the other times when he called me by the wrong name. I still struggle with the reality of that particular moment—was it a trance, or was I in a dream?

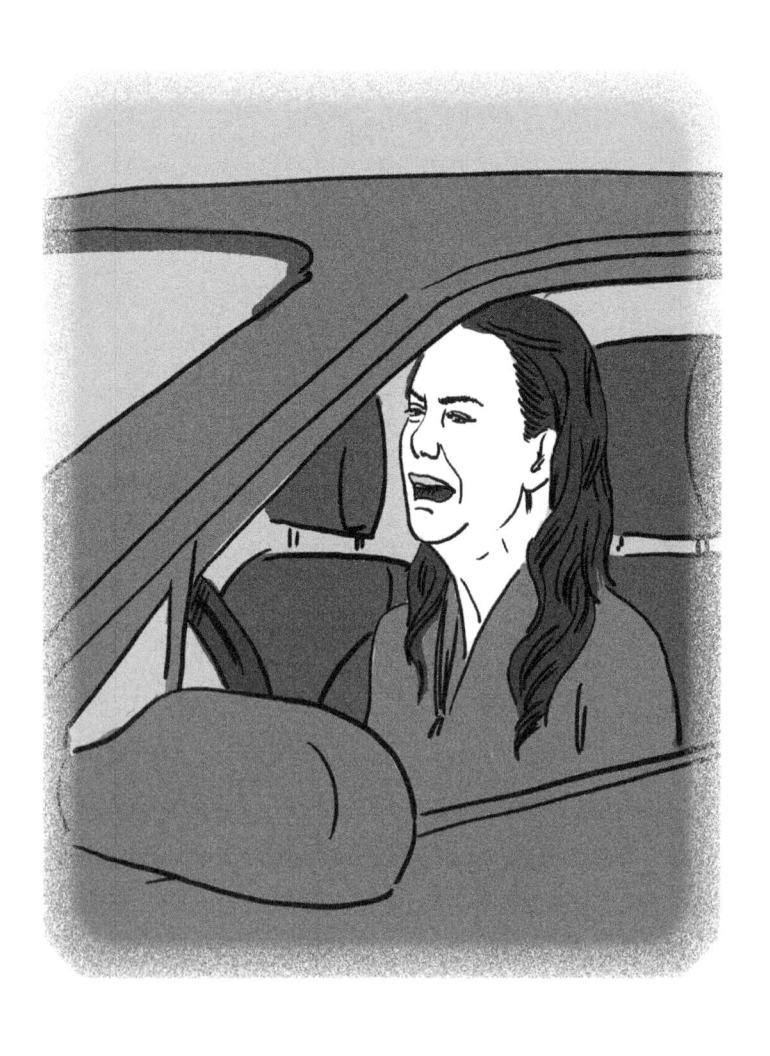

The Day My Dad Forgot Me

During breakfast, Dad started to ask me questions. He asked if I was his niece. I thought he was joking. I replied that I was not his niece. Dad insisted I was his niece. I repeated that I was not his niece, and I told him that I was, in fact, his daughter. He chuckled and emphatically replied that he did not have a daughter. I was shocked.

Unfortunately, the time came when Dad couldn't recognize many faces and had zero concept of age. He thought Mom was in her twenties and looked gorgeous, which pleased her to no end. He thought Leslie was in her thirties and looked nice in a plain sort of way. But he had never addressed me in any way other than the occasional, "How ya doing, Sir," which didn't really bother me because once I responded that I was his daughter, Lindsey, he would then respond with "Oh, yes, of course."

This time was different. I knew that he did not recognize me as his daughter at all. I also knew that I was lost to him forever. I had been wiped clean of his memory bank. Painfully, I was the first one to be totally forgotten. Or, at least it seemed that way.

I asked myself, *Why couldn't it have been Leslie?* Leslie would have been fine with it. Leslie would not have taken the slightest offense. Her rationale in dealing with Duane's illness was largely practical. She never took it personally. Or at least she never gave me that impression.

"It's not personal," she would always say, before shortly adding, "he has a disease that robs memories." Leslie has the strength of practicality and logic that I lacked at the time.

But none of what Leslie said made a hoot of a difference to me. *I am his flesh and blood daughter! How could he forget ME!!* I became hysterical, frenzied, and agitated. I couldn't come to terms with it. I had to call Mom at work and tell her. "Dad has officially forgotten me, and I can't deal with it, so I am bringing him to you at work."

Mom managed a medical clinic that was not totally conducive for dropping off family members who needed care, but nonetheless, she agreed and said it was okay to bring him to the clinic.

Leslie arrived at about the same time I did, and, again, she reminded me that it is not personal. "Really, Leslie?" I asked. "Well, it is definitely personal to me," I added.

I dropped him off and headed back home as quickly as possible, laughing and crying uncontrollably at the same time. *How could my own father forget me?* I spent two days in bed before I could wrap my head around what had happened. It was later that Leslie confessed to me that Dad had also forgotten her a few years earlier. Dad thought Leslie was the average-looking, thirty-year-old housekeeper.

Although what Leslie confessed was mildly amusing, it didn't help matters nor did it lessen the pain of being forgotten forever by my dad.

"YOU ONLY KNOW YOURSELF BECAUSE OF YOUR MEMORIES."

—ANDREA GILLIS

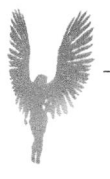

CHAPTER ELEVEN

BREAKING NEWS – LESLIE

Duane had been the ultimate ad-man. He did it all—television, print ads, live events, and news stories. He made stories happen for his clients. Unfortunately, the tables had turned, and it was Duane who was now in the news.

Breaking News: 69-year-old man with dementia is missing. He stands 5'8" 150 lbs with silver hair. He was last seen in the Kirkland area wearing a blue polo shirt with khaki slacks. Here is his picture. Please call ## ### #### if you see him.

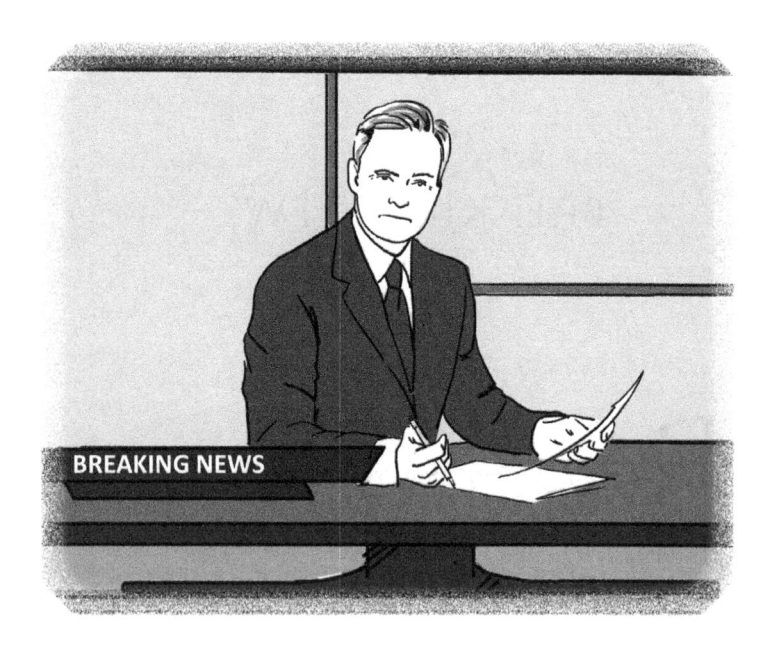

Breaking News

Earlier that morning, Mom had called to inform me that Duane had been missing since the previous night. Mom and Lindsey had canvassed the neighborhood searching for Duane, but as night fell and the temperature became unbearable they went back home. He did not have a coat, the temperature was below 40 degrees, and it was raining. I knew better than to ask anyone how this could have happened and why on heaven's earth they did not contact me earlier. People with dementia are escape artists.

I explained to my husband what my mother had told me, and we began our own search party. After hours of searching around, we still could not find him. My kids and their friends got involved too, by asking people in the neighborhood if they had seen an elderly man looking lost. We created flyers to post. After endless hours with no sign of Duane, we headed back to Mom's house to wait. Seconds felt like minutes. Minutes felt like hours. Hours felt like days.

Finally, we heard a knock on the door. When I opened the front door, there was Duane, chipper as he could be, with a couple of new friends, aka police officers. Duane was clean and perfectly dry.

The first thing he said was, "Hello, ladies," and then he proceeded to cordially introduce us to his newfound mates. Duane had no idea where he had been or what had happened, but the police officers told us that a nice couple had dropped him off at a hotel. Apparently, Duane had told the hotel personnel that he had an important business meeting there and was waiting for his clients to arrive. After several hours of waiting, the hotel management figured out that something wasn't quite right and they called the police.

Nevertheless, there were still several hours unaccounted for. Yet, he here was—clean and dry. We all decided that the nice couple must have taken him in, kept him warm, and fed him before bringing him to the hotel. The hotel manager said that Duane had told him that after his business meeting, he was traveling to Canada.

"Canada? What's with Canada?" I said out loud because Duane had never been to Canada.

"EVERY DAY I WAS A NEW FRIEND TO HIM."
—LESLIE BIRKLAND

CHAPTER TWELVE
DIAPER DUTY – LESLIE

It had been exactly six years since Duane was diagnosed with dementia. My mind was boggled by all the information available on dementia websites, laying out its stages of progression.

Many articles say dementia is irreversible and incurable, but with an early diagnosis and proper care, the progression of some forms of dementia can be managed and slowed down. The cognitive decline that accompanies dementia does not happen all at once. Its progression can be divided into distinct, identifiable stages. In the first stage, there is no impairment.

During this stage, dementia's disease is hard or near impossible to detect, and there are no memory problems or other symptoms to confirm the presence of dementia. It becomes worse as it progresses until there is an extremely severe decline.

The time frame varies for each individual suffering with the disease. You can remain in stage one for years. Run a business, drive a car, and so on. The downside of this stage is they tend to make poor business decisions that can affect entire families and employees.

In our case, our hopes held us hostage, in constant denial, believing that God would fully restore Duane to his former self. I know that God listens and answers every prayer, *No Exceptions*. It just may not be the answer we want.

When Duane progressed to an advanced stage, he was 85% confined to bed. A nice hospital bed smack dab in the middle of the living room. He softly spoke often about seeing angels. While that was beautiful, he also talked about seeing the entire Husky football team practicing outside in the yard. Incredible! God and football. That can only sound like Duane.

Diaper Duty

Mom kept Duane clean and fresh. It was not easy, and, most times, it was a big struggle. She is a small-sized woman, and it took everything out of her to make Duane's life as comfortable as possible. He could barely walk. It was more like a shuffle. On rare occasions, he could get up to use the toilet on his own. However, most of the time Mom had to assist him. He wore big man diapers, and sometimes he would rip them off. Unfortunately, the cleanup was fully on Mom. I pitied Mom every time I saw her do this, knowing the toll it was taking on her. So, I advised her that it was time to put Duane in a nursing facility where they could take around-the-clock care of him. Mom was having none of it. She wasn't ready to take that step. She believed that nursing homes are where people go to die, and she didn't believe it was time for that.

Mom rarely left home. I would pick her up when Duane was in a deep sleep, and together we would rush to the grocery store or the pharmacy. We had it perfectly timed, so we would be gone for less than 20 minutes. One particular day, as we were approaching the house from a quick errand, we saw Duane. He was walking slowly down the lane, wearing only a diaper and hugging his blanket.

We could not believe our eyes. It was the saddest, most pitiful thing I had ever witnessed. A once vibrant businessman, devoted husband, and caring father demoted to the role of a mere toddler. It was so painful to watch.

The following week, Duane's primary care doctor came for a house visit to evaluate Duane. He told us it was time for Duane to go to a nursing home facility. He also gave us the number for hospice. Mom was very scared because of the uncertainties and the unknowns that can be encountered with Social Security and Medicare. I wondered, *How can she afford to place him in a nursing home and still afford her household bills?* I told Mom the best thing to do was to simply call the Social Security office and find out.

In the meantime, we ordered a bracelet for Duane that had the medical alert symbol as well as Mom's phone number on it. This was something we should have done much earlier.

HE OFTEN SPOKE OF SEEING ANGELS.
ONE THING IS FOR CERTAIN,
THE ANGELS SAW HIM."

—JUDITH DENHOF

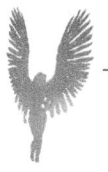

CHAPTER THIRTEEN
SUPPORT GROUPS – LESLIE

Everything turned out fine with Social Security and Medicare. A few months after the doctor's recommendation, Duane was placed in a nursing home. He was treated with kindness and respect. He was bathed every day and hand-fed each meal. He managed to use the heels of his feet to maneuver himself around the circular complex in a wheelchair. Evidently, he still enjoyed circles.

Mom would drive to see him every single day. She would talk to him about what was going on with the family as she felt it was important to talk to him as if

Daughters of Dementia

he understood everything she was saying. Sometimes, he would laugh out loud at something she thought he thought was particularly amusing. This gave us a faint sense of hope. Part of Duane was still in there, we just knew it.

Mom joined a dementia support group. She strongly believed that it would help her to be with other people who shared some of her experiences. People who identified with her struggles emotionally. I was totally in support of her decision. But the reality was, however, not at all what she expected.

She went to her first meeting hoping to meet people who would really empathize with her, but alas, that was the first and last time she went to this group. It was horrifying! She came home in tears. Tears for the caregivers and tears for the ones with dementia.

Their stories were beyond belief. Women tying their loved ones to chairs. Beating them to submission. Most of the families were pissed off and angry that they had to take care of someone who wouldn't listen or take instructions. One man was furious that his wife stopped making him breakfast. She had

Support Groups

been making him breakfast for 40 years, and one day, she suddenly stopped. It didn't matter that she had dementia, he was hungry and wanted breakfast. Another man forced his wife to have sex with him every night in hopes that she would remember him. She was *his* wife, he explained, so he didn't consider it rape for a moment. It was appalling beyond reason. He confessed that she would scream and cry the whole time. He said that he hoped sex would somehow jog her memory and that it would bring them closer together again.

Not one person in the group, not even the group organizers, stood up to tell these people that what they were doing was tantamount to abuse or criminal activity and that they had to stop it. NOT ONE.

I kept wondering what would have happened if I had been there. I am pretty certain all hell would have broken loose. How could these people think for a moment they were equipped to be caretakers? It takes understanding, research, talking to doctors, and most importantly, being aware that you cannot bully dementia out of a person. Just like you cannot bully cancer out of a person.

Mom found solace with another group. A group that helped people who choose to be caregivers, and to learn the tools to cope and assist their loved one.

Whether or not a person has a loved one with dementia's, we must all know that dementia is a disease and we cannot control it. We must treat anyone who has dementia's with dignity.

It has five stages:

- Stage 1: No impairment. The patient has no problems.
- Stage 2: Questionable impairment. The patient begins to have some difficulty but can still function independently.
- Stage 3: Mild impairment. The patient has obvious, but still mild, difficulty with daily activities.
- Stage 4: Moderate impairment. The patient needs help with caring for himself or herself as well as with carrying out daily activities.
- Stage 5: Severe impairment. Patients are unable to function independently.

CHAPTER FOURTEEN

HOSPICE – LESLIE

Duane had been in the care of the nursing home for two years. The director called Mom and said it was time for her to contact Duane's doctor and discuss hospice. Hospice is a wonderful organization that focuses on the patient's physical, emotional, and spiritual needs at the end of life. Hospice services are available only when the patient's doctor believes the patient has six months or less to live. Duane's doctor confirmed that it was indeed time, and we had to get everything in order. By that time, Duane was unable to eat, talk, walk, or hold his head up by himself. He was a shell of the strong, vibrant man he once had been. A shadow of his former self. He would just stare, glassy eyed for long lengths of time, looking at absolutely nothing.

All of us wanted to believe that he was still in there, listening to each and every word that we spoke, but somehow, we had to come to terms with the fact that his mind was gone. It was one of the most heart-wrenching moments of my life. After eight years of being the pragmatic one in the family, I finally cracked.

I could see it was the beginning of the end for Duane, and, yes, I felt guilty for being secretly happy. Happy for him, happy that his suffering was to end, if not today, then soon. But still, it was all too much for me to bear, and I cracked. I called my kids and made them promise to never let me get to the same point as Grandpa Duane. I mean, not even close to this point. I don't want to be the lady running around the neighborhood naked with my bra on my head. Whatever it takes, I told them.

Witnessing this horrid, dreadful, unforgiving disease finally got to me. After the tragic drowning of their own father, my kids didn't even want to discuss

Hospice

my wishes about the end of my life. However, they finally agreed, if only to pacify my grief over Duane. After all, it wasn't about me, and I had to come to grips with myself to help Mom and Lindsey in any way possible.

Duane remained in a semi-comatose state for five more months. Then came "The Call." The dreaded call from Hospice. The nurse said, "It's time. He is actively dying, and it could be a day or even minutes."

By the time I arrived with my friend Ralph, Mom and Lindsey were already there, sitting next to Duane as he lay motionless in his bed. The nurses, who had grown quite fond of Duane, had tears in their eyes. They would stop by his room every ten minutes to check on Duane and ask if we needed anything. Mom's dear friend and pastor arrived for prayer. Duane had what the nurses and doctor referred to as the death rattle. He would take in a deep breath and sputter out as he exhaled.

We were all tired. We took turns staying with Duane, so each of us could take a rest on the grassy area outside in the courtyard. My friend Ralph had to leave, so when Mom's dear friend was about to leave, Mom suggested that I should go as well and get some rest. I was tired, but so was everyone. But, Mom insisted I should leave, so I went. Twenty-five minutes later, Mom called me on my cell phone to say Duane had passed away.

Lindsey was alone with her father as he took his last breath.

I told her we would turn around and come back, but Mom said the funeral home was on the way, so it was unnecessary.

Months after Duane's passing, Mom and I were going through Duane's personal papers. We noticed a calendar under some newspapers. All the months and days in the calendar were empty. With one extraordinary exception. Marked on the very day my husband had passed away in a tragic accident, Duane had written, "Always Remember this Day!" We determined it had to have been written prior to the accident. Mom and I looked at one another in utter amazement. Perhaps Duane really did see the angels he spoke about. We both got chills and wished we had paid more attention to Duane's utterances, as we believe they very well were prophetic messages from heaven.

> "WE'RE REALLY A COMPOSITE
> OF OUR LIFE EXPERIENCES –
> MEMORY LAYERED UPON MEMORY
> AND ALZHEIMER'S STEALS THAT AWAY."
>
> —MERYL COMER

CHAPTER FIFTEEN

THE DAY MY DAD DIED – LINDSEY

Mom and I were driving to the nursing home to visit Dad. The day before, he had appeared extremely pale and his breathing was slower than normal. His eyes were shut tight, and he barely moved a muscle. As we approached the facility, Mom received a call from the director of the nursing home saying it was imminent and we should come now. There had been many times when we thought it was his last day. So, we were not certain. Not certain until we saw him. There was no question that this fateful day was to be the day. The day my father would be with God

Daughters of Dementia

the Father. Moments later, Leslie arrived with her friend Ralph. Leslie asked the nurse if this was for sure. The nurse spoke softly and said, "Yes, we are certain. Please prepare yourselves."

Mom knew that this was going to be the final day. Duane's breathing continued to labor. The nurse explained that this is called the death rattle. He would gasp for breath and exhale in what seemed like stuttering. A couple of Mom's closest friends arrived for moral support. We all sat there lined up in metal folding chairs on one side of his bed. We all prayed, but for the most part there was little conversation. Leslie and Ralph left to get food for everyone. They came back with McDonald's hamburgers. So, there we all sat, eating McDonald's, staring at Dad in silence. A few hours later, Leslie was tired and left. About 20 minutes later, my dad stopped breathing. Mom was outside in the courtyard. I went to her and said, "I think he's gone."

The nurse confirmed that Duane had indeed passed on. It was a surreal moment. He was actually gone. His mind had left us long ago, but now his body had given up the fight. My dad was 75.

CHAPTER SIXTEEN

FRIENDS OF DEMENTIA – LESLIE

My dear friend Liz called me and wanted to talk about dementia. Her mother had always been a difficult woman, but now it was much more than her daily complaints. Liz shared that her mom, who typically called her once or twice a day, was calling her every 20 minutes. Liz's mom told her the government was after her and people were spying on her. Her mom would go to the bank and withdraw all her money, only to open a new account at a different bank. The next week she would put all her money in yet another bank.

Liz did not live in the same state as her mother. It was all on Liz's sister Corrina to manage this turn of events. Liz felt sorry for Corrina having to take on most of the burden, especially since their mother thought Corrina was stealing from her. I told Liz to immediately get a Durable Power of Attorney. In this case, Liz's mother was very much the person she had always been with the exception of severe delusions. She refused to sign a Power of Attorney, and Corrina eventually had to get a court order, which was a pretty lengthy process.

It was difficult for Corrina to find a care facility that would take their mother. Not all nursing homes take on dementia patients. Her delusions were constant, and she was hostile and violent, so she needed a more intensive level of care. Eventually, Corrina was able to find a place with a dementia wing that would accept her mother as a patient. The phone calls to Liz remained relentless even from the nursing home. Liz had to make the sad decision to block her own mom.

Another dear friend, Dee, called me, frantic about her grandfather. He was 80, and her grandmother was 74. Grandpa had been diagnosed with dementia a few years earlier. Grandpa remembered most of the family members, including Dee. When family would come to visit, he would whisper, "Help! That old lady is keeping me hostage here."

Grandma explained that he would try to run away every day to escape the house. She said she had to pull him off their fence. Dee noticed that Grandpa had a lot of bruises all over his body. Her grandma would explain that he fell down or off the fence. It turned out that Grandma was beating the living hell out of him every day. Neighbors had to call the authorities to report disturbances over at Grandma and Grandpa's house.

I told Dee to have Grandma call Social Security as well as Medicare to get Grandpa placed in a safe environment. In the meantime, I advised her to tell Grandma to get large black rugs and put them at the front and back doors. I had read that people with dementia do not recognize a black rug as a floor mat, but rather as a deep hole. Nursing homes have also taken to using black carpets to deter escapees.

Well, the black carpet worked; however, he died a month later.

CHAPTER SEVENTEEN
IMAGINE – LESLIE

After Duane passed on, Lindsey and I have dedicated our lives to Dementia Awareness, Dementia Abuse, and helping those who have a loved one with this misunderstood disease. Our father, Duane, prior to dementia had a mellow temperament. He was, in fact, a calm individual. After his diagnosis, he did not ever get violent and was happy to meet new people. Everyone was NEW people to him, even us at a certain point. However, that is not always the case.

Take a moment and imagine. Imagine you are home alone watching television. A strange man walks into your house. You have never seen this man in your life. Then he starts screaming at you to stop talking. You were not talking in the first place. Next, this man demands that you go with him in his car. What do you do?

I would probably call the police or grab something near me to use a weapon to protect myself from this intruder. I might just run and keep running. This is what dementia looks like from the sufferer's point of view. They DO NOT know you! You are a stranger. You cannot make dementia go away by yelling. I have said this countless times, and I'll keep saying it until everyone understands it's the truth. A person with dementia doesn't know she is asking the same question over and over again. In her mind, the 100th time is the first time she's asking a question.

Demanding a person with dementia to "act the way we want them to" would be like demanding a blind person to see again. You cannot ask a blind person to see by demanding he just look harder.

Dementia cannot be bullied out of someone. It is a disease! It is not a reason to be embarrassed. It is also important at some point to let family, friends, and neighbors know that your loved one has dementia. Don't put your loved ones in danger because you are afraid people may think less of them or that telling others about their dementia would somehow diminish the great person they had once been.

Below are some resources that can help:

- Alzhiemer's Foundation – www.alzfdn.org

- Alzhiemer's Society of America – www.DementiaSociety.org

- Alzhiemer's Association – www.Alz.org

- Dementia's Research – www.dementias.net

- Family Caregiver Alliance – www.caregiver.org

- National Hospice and Palliative Care Organization – www.nhpco.org

"WE REMEMBER THEIR LOVE WHEN THEY CAN NO LONGER REMEMBER."
—UNKNOWN

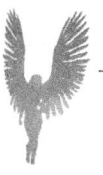

CHAPTER EIGHTEEN

DEMENTIA OR JUST GETTING OLD - LESLIE

On the day Duane was officially diagnosed with dementia, Mom was justifiably distressed. But it did explain a lot of things about his odd behavior. Duane, on the other hand, did not fully understand what it meant. He happily took all the tests. Mom said he was obliging and, of course, funny. The neurologist told Mom that Duane was the most intelligent man he had ever tested. He also said directly to Duane that after years of taking care of his family it was time to let the family take care of him. The doctor then told Mom that anything Duane does or does not do, is not his fault. Those words held strong for Mom as she took care of Duane for the next 10 years.

Once they arrived home, Duane started to write and write. He wrote about his love for family and how important it is to appreciate life every day. He continued to write that he was dying and that his death was imminent. There was no mention of what the cause of his imminent death was, yet it was soon. It was a beautiful letter that he tucked away in a drawer and soon forgot all about it. Duane never knew he had dementia.

Mom and I often spoke about "what if's"—what if one of us got dementia, what would we do? Would we even know? Every time either of us would forget something, we would think, *Oh, no! Maybe I have dementia*. After all these years, I do know one thing. If you think you have dementia, you probably don't. We all age, and with aging comes normal forgetfulness. Memory lapses are normal with older adults and are not considered a warning sign of dementia. Forgetting where you left your eyeglasses or keys is normal. Calling your grandchild three different names before you get it right is normal. Walking into a room and forgetting why you entered at all, is normal. Having the answer to a question on the tip of your tongue and then it is gone, is normal.

Mom and I made a pact that if either of us are diagnosed with dementia we would let the other know. Which of course makes no sense because people with dementia do not know they have dementia, even if they are told a hundred times. But dementia makes no sense, so we are keeping to our pact.

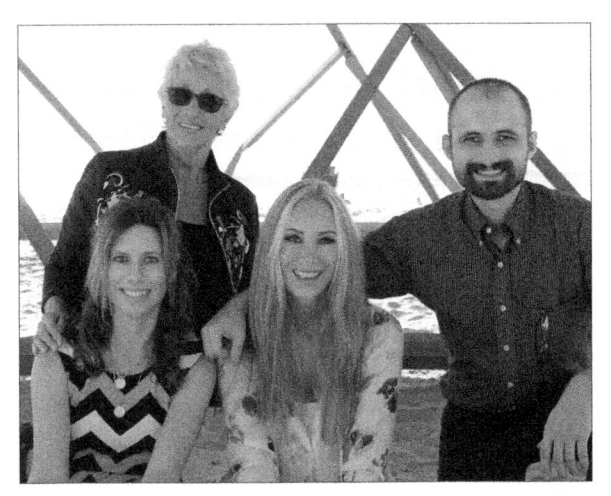

Us today, visiting one of Duane's favorites beaches in California. Lindsey, mom, Leslie and Leslie's son, Nick

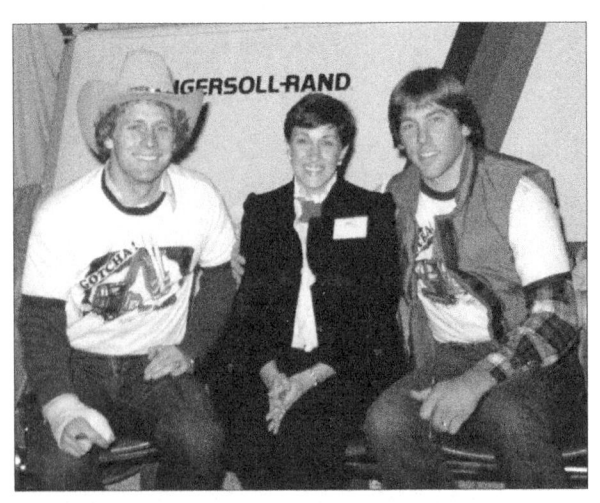

One of Duane's advertising campaigns with Mom sitting between Seattle Seahawks super stars, Steve Largent and Jim Zorn

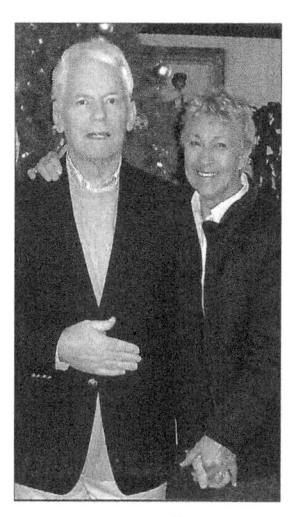

*Duane and Mom
Christmas 2013*

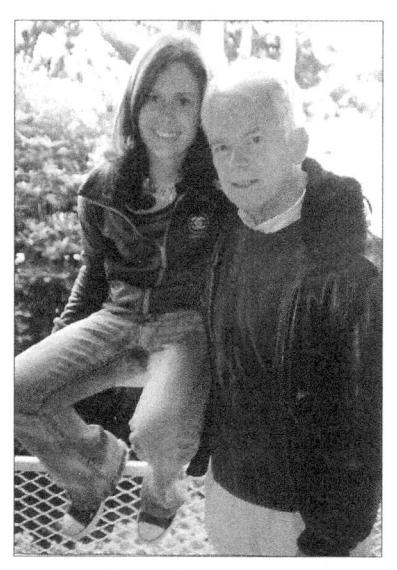

*Lindsey's favorite picture
with her dad*

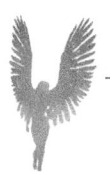

ABOUT THE AUTHORS

LESLIE BIRKLAND

Leslie Birkland is renowned for being the woman who went from welfare to the reality hit show, *Big Rich Texas*. She attributes her modeling career to her stepfather, Duane. If it were not for him, there would have been no career. Modeling provided much more then posing for pictures and parading down the catwalk. She has traveled internationally for modeling assignments on a number of occasions.

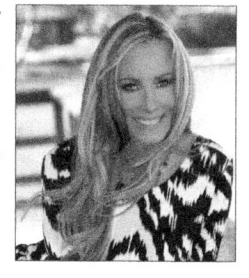

Being on magazine covers and getting paid for it was nice, but it was immersing herself in diverse cultures around the world that changed her life and gave her an appreciation for all people.

Growing up poor and understanding the value of saving money, Leslie was able to pay her own tuition and ultimately obtained a BA in Communications in 1985. Recently, she completed a program and is now a certified Wellness Coach, specializing in Holistic Medicine in hopes of finding natural ways to slow down the dementia spiral.

Currently, Leslie travels between her two homes in Canyon Lake, California, and Seattle, Washington. She is the mother of three grown boys.

Website: LattesWithLeslie.com
Facebook: @lesliebirkland
Twitter: @lesliebirkland

About the Authors

LINDSEY DENHOF

Lindsey Denhof is a singer/songwriter and is writing songs in memory of her father. She attended Central College in Washington State with an emphasis on the Arts. In 2006, she graduated from the City Church Intern program. Currently, Lindsey resides in San Diego. She is an active member at City Church of San Diego and is one of the Worship team leaders. In her spare time, Lindsey can be found at her art studio creating paintings with fingernail polish. Her art can be seen in many art galleries throughout Southern California.

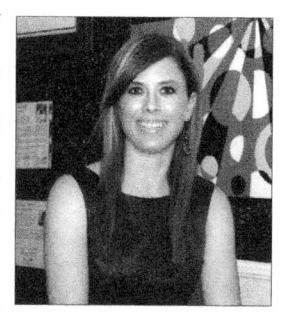

Website: Fyoom-art.com

Made in the USA
Middletown, DE
20 August 2019